Graves Disease

A Guide for Patients

Andrew McLaren FRCS

Graves Disease

The Thyroid Gland in Normal Health

Overactive Thyroid

Diagnosis of Graves Disease

    Symptoms

    Physical Signs

    Biochemical Tests

    Radiological Tests

Medical Treatment of Graves Disease

Definitive Treatment of Graves Disease

Radio-iodine for Graves Disease

Surgery for Graves Disease

Graves Disease

Graves' disease is a disease of the body's immune system.

The immune system for reasons that are unclear can produce antibodies which are able to attach themselves to receptors on the surface of thyroid cells.

These antibodies act as *thyroid stimulating antibodies* and cause the thyroid cells to produce more thyroid hormone. The thyroid gland may also enlarge.

The condition is more common in women and can run in families to some extent as there are particular genetic factors which make it more likely to occur.

The commonest group is young women (20 to 40 years of age) although the disease can occur in men it is much less common.

Graves disease was described by Dr Robert James Graves (1796-1853) in a monograph on the subject published in 1835 and entitled:

"A Newly Observed Affection of the Thyroid Gland in Females"

The Thyroid Gland in Normal Health

The thyroid gland produces several hormones:

Thyroxine – T4

Tri-iodothyronine – T3

Calcitonin

Thyroxine and tri-iodothyronine are stored in the thyroid. The storage is done in colloid jelly which is another substance made by the thyroid.

Within this colloid the hormones are bound to thyroglobulin.

The thyroid gland contains a very large store of thyroid hormone sufficient for several weeks.

T4 and T3 are released by the thyroid gland into the blood stream. The control of this process is incredibly tight and regulated by a further hormone (thyroid stimulating hormone) made by the pituitary gland in the brain.

The control process is tight because the thyroid system is so crucial to normal health.

Human beings cannot grow and develop without thyroid hormone. This is why babies are checked within days of birth to ensure their thyroid gland is present and functioning.

Some babies are born without a thyroid gland and this results in poor mental and physical development with a thick protruding tongue being one of the characteristic features of the condition termed "cretinism".

T3 is the key thyroid hormone and the bit that does all the work in the cells of the body.

A tiny amount of T3 is actually made by the thyroid. The bulk of it is produced in the tissues where it is actually needed and comes from breaking down T4. This process is known as peripheral conversion.

The bloodstream effectively acts as a massive store of thyroid hormone because T4 has a long half-life taking 7 days for the level of T4 in the blood to drop by 50% even if no more is made.

When the body senses thyroid hormone levels are dropping the pituitary gland makes more TSH to increase production and release.

TSH increases thyroid hormone production and also enlargement of the thyroid gland. Reduced TSH levels lead to shrinkage of the thyroid gland.

Calcitonin

For the purposes of this book we wont consider calcitonin as it has no impact on the thyroid system.

Calcitonin is part of the control system for calcium levels in the body and entirely unconnected to the thyroid hormones.

Overactive Thyroid

An overactive thyroid or hyperthyroidism occurs in women and men but is ten times more common in women (27 cases per 1000 women).

There are a number of causes of hyperthyroidism and these are listed below for the sake of completeness but Graves disease is by far the most common:

Graves disease
Toxic multi-nodular goitre
Toxic solitary nodule
Thyroiditis

A whole host of symptoms are caused by the excess thyroid hormones circulating in the blood. These include:

Fast heart rate - tachycardia
Palpitations
Weight loss
Sweating
Feeling hot
Nervousness
Irritability
Diarrhoea
Irregular periods
Hair loss

Tiredness and lethargy

One of the most interesting features of hyperthyroidism is that most patients will feel tired and run down even though one would expect them to feel more energy from the excess of thyroid hormone.

The simplest way of explaining this is that the body has a disease process going on and therefore its not surprising people don't feel right. However, clearly it is more complex than that.

There is certainly an impact from disturbed sleep which most patients experience and also the overactive state leads to a drive to do more which can't be sustained.

Even when the disease is brought under control by medication many patients still feel run down. Fortunately this resolves with definitive treatment.

Diagnosis of Graves Disease

Symptoms

Physical Signs

You may see signs of weight loss, anxiety and sweatiness.

The hands may show a fine tremor particularly when the arms are outstretched (due to overactivity of the sympathetic nervous system). The palms of the hands can become erythematous (reddened) and can feel warm and sweaty.

The pulse rate is usually elevated but may slip into atrial fibrillation (an irregular heart beat).

The eyes classically show a protrusion of the eyeball (exophthalmos). This may be obvious and is characterized by the white of the eye (sclera) being visible above the eyeball when it is normally covered by the eyelid.

Exophthalmos only occurs in Graves disease so if present establishes the diagnosis.

It is caused by the antibody of Graves disease attacking the soft tissues within the orbital cavity. This causes them to become inflamed and swollen reducing the space in this boney pocket and pushing the eyeball out as a consequence.

Biochemical Tests

T4 levels will be elevated

TSH will be suppressed

Thyroid TSH receptor antibody levels may be elevated

Radiological Tests

Radioactive iodine uptake scans can be used to assess the overactive thyroid gland.

They should only rarely be required to assess Graves disease – as most cases can be diagnosed from clinical signs and blood tests.

However, if there is doubt about the diagnosis and particularly if there are no physical signs of Graves one should be done.

The most important diagnosis to exclude is a solitary toxic nodule. This condition is easy to treat with either radioactive iodine or surgery once the overactive thyroid has been brought under control with medication.

A toxic nodule will not improve with longterm anti-thyroid medication and patients therefore need to be identified and offered definitive treatment of some sort at an early stage.

Medical Treatment for Graves Disease

All patients with Graves disease will need treatment to bring the disease under control and hopefully get rid of all or most of the symptoms.

This will allow time to investigate and confirm the diagnosis if required and then to plan further management.

Medical treatment requires the use of anti-thyroid drugs and two are used in clinical practice:

Carbimazole (CBZ)

Propylthiouracil (PTU)

There really isn't too much to choose between these two drugs. They both work by interfering with the way in which iodine is incorporated into thyroid hormone and effectively block thyroid hormone production.

Carbimazole is more commonly used in the UK although in the USA most doctors prescribe propythiouracil.

Propylthiouracil is used in pregnant women as the drug is less able to cross the placenta and affect the developing foetus than carbimazole.

Traditionally patients would be given a starting dose which is relatively high – CBZ 10-20mg three times daily or PTU 100mg three times daily. Most patients will find that they feel better quickly and blood tests will show thyroid function coming under control.

Once the disease is controlled the drug dose can be progressively reduced and in an ideal world get down to a low maintenance dose where the disease is kept under control and normal thyroid function maintained. The hope is that the tablets will result in a permanent remission of the disease which burns itself out during the drug treatment period.

In general, once this controlled state is reached patients are advised to continue taking the tablets for 12-18 months before stopping them.

At this point it is worth mentioning that not everyone is lucky enough for the disease to burn itself out during the treatment maintenance phase.

A large number of patients find that the disease comes back. Indeed studies show that around 40% will relapse in the first year off drugs and a further 20% in subsequent years – so in reality fewer than half are completely cured.

This is pretty shocking news for many patients as having relapsed they will then have to restart the higher drug doses to bring the disease back under control and then once stable consider which definitive treatment to have as clearly tablets wont work permanently.

Increasingly I am seeing patients opting in the first phase of treatment to have a definitive procedure – either radioactive iodine or surgery – to avoid this relapse issue.

These figures of course only relate to those patients who can be "cured" with tablets. There are a significant number where tablets will never bring the disease fully under control – these patients will need to come to surgery as they cant have radio-active iodine as a definitive option (see RAI section).

Side Effects of Antithyroid Medication

Minor side effects include – itching (pruritis), nausea, mild joint pains and skin rashes.

The most serious side effect which all should be warned to take seriously is the potential effect of either drug on the bone marrow.

For reasons which aren't clear both anti-thyroid drugs can effectively wipe out the immune system by stopping the production of white blood cells which are crucial to defence (agranulocytosis).

Agranulocytosis can occur early on or even after years of taking the drugs hence the desire not to use these as long term medications.

All patients should be clearly advised that if they get a sore throat and fever the medication should be stopped and medical advice sought.

If agranulocytosis does occur it generally resolves rapidly once the medication is stopped but clearly the same tablet cannot be restarted and a number of patients will find they also then react to the alternate tablet.

As a result it is pretty common for this group to be referred urgently for surgery.

Beta-adrenergic blockers

These drugs such as propranolol can reduce many of the symptoms of the symptoms of Graves disease – particularly those that affect the cardiovascular system e.g., palpitations and tachycardia.

The drugs also have a beneficial effect of reducing the conversion of T4 the less active thyroid hormone into the more active T3 so further boosting the benefit of their use.

Many doctors use them as a routine adjunct to treatment.

Alternatively and probably more sensibly the drugs are reserved for patients with palpitations or for those who are not well controlled and are being prepared for surgery.

Thyroid Crisis or Storm

Thyroid crisis is rare.

It is a potentially life-threatening condition that usually occurs in patients who have just undergone surgery for Graves disease.

Hormones released by manipulation of the gland result in an acute and very severe thyrotoxic state after surgery.

Clinically this results in a number of symptoms:

- tachycardia
- high temperature
- restlessness
- confusional state
- vomiting
- diarrhea

Treatment is by giving propyl-thiouracil and iodine regularly along with careful administration of propranolol along with careful supportive measures usually meaning admission to an intensive care unit.

It is for this reason that most surgeons are obsessed with ensuring patients thyroid condition is properly controlled before undertaking surgery and quite rightly have no hesitation in cancelling surgery for patients who are not controlled.

Clearly there are some cases where surgery needs to be undertaken on an emergency basis and this can be done safely with careful liaison with a medical endocrinologist and engaging help from an anaesthetist with an interest in thyroid surgery.

Definitive Treatment of Graves Disease

For some definitive treatment is required after relapse of Graves off tablets, a failure to ever get the disease under full control and for a minority it is part of their treatment choice from the start.

There are only two definitive treatment options:

1. Radioactive iodine

2. Total thyroidectomy surgery

Sometimes patients are keen to stay on anti-thyroid drugs longterm. This is rarely a good option as most people are not on top form with Graves disease even if supposedly controlled by tablets and the side-effects are unpredictable and can be serious.

Radio-iodine for Graves Disease

Iodine works to treat Graves disease as iodine is an integral component of thyroid hormones and is taken into thyroid cells as they attempt to manufacture thyroid hormone.

As a result of this and the fact that thyroid cells are the only cells in the body that use iodine and therefore take it into themselves radioactive iodine can be used to target and selectively kill them.

The iodine used is ^{131}I and is used in a typical dose of 555 megabecquerels (MBq).

Whilst this is a radiation based treatment the dose required is small due to the concentration of its effect within the thyroid. Many studies have been done which show that the risks of this treatment are extremely low and there is no evidence to suggest of harm from the radiation.

In particular large studies that have followed treated patients for many years show no increase in risk of cancer.

In the UK the use of radio-active iodine is generally avoided in women who intend to have children within 1 year or those with thyroid eye disease. It can only be used in patients where the thyroid system has been brought under control by medication.

In the UK despite the evidence of safety there is a public perception that radiation based treatments should be avoided which is widely held.

This contrasts with the US where the treatment is extensively used and is even used in children.

Radio-active iodine treatment side-effects:

1. Treatment failure

   Dependent on the dose of radioactive iodine used and the size of the thyroid the treatment may not completely destroy the thyroid resulting in the overactive state returning. A further dose of radioactive iodine is needed in up to 25% of patients.

2. Local discomfort

As the thyroid gland is destroyed it becomes inflamed and sore. This may be evident with local discomfort including a sore throat which generally lasts a few days

3. Increase in thyrotoxic symptoms

   Cell breakdown results in release of thyroid hormones and may cause an increase in thyrotoxic symptoms. The radioactive iodine treatment should always be covered with anti-thyroid mediation and beta blockers may help.

4. Hypothyroidism

   Most patients after radioactive iodine will end up becoming underactive in respect of thyroid function (60% at 1 year post treatment).

   For those that do not become underactive careful long term surveillance is required with thyroxine replacement as required.

5. Thyroid eye disease

Thyroid eye disease can be made worse with radioactive iodine. Sometimes the impact can be reduced with the use of oral steroid tablets however the damage to vision can be permanent.

For this reason many endocrinologists are uncomfortable about recommending iodine therapy when eye disease is present favouring surgery as a definitive treatment.

Surgery for Graves Disease

Thyroid surgery for Graves disease is a safe procedure nowadays and results in the patient rapidly becoming normal in terms of thyroid function.

The key reasons for undertaking thyroid surgery are:

1. Relapse of Graves disease after a period of drug treatment

2. Severe thyrotoxicosis which is not controlled with tablets

3. Thyrotoxicosis which doesn't come under control with tablets – often this is due to poor compliance by the patient with their drug regime

4. Large thyroid goitre – a large thyroid due to Graves disease will shrink to some extent with radio-active iodine but may remain sizeable and symptomatic and these patients often require more than one course of radioactive iodine

The surgery for Graves disease should be a total thyroidectomy removing all thyroid tissue.

There is no role for the now discredited operation of sub-total thyroidectomy.

It is worth considering why sub-total thyroidectomy was suggested as a surgical option as this helps understand why it is a poor option.

The aim of the subtotal surgery was to leave a remnant of thyroid tissue behind – judged very carefully – to preserve normal thyroid function and remove the need for thyroid replacement with tablets.

The remnant left was the upper pole of the thyroid on one or both sides of the neck. Thus providing a potential secondary benefit of aiding preservation of the superior parathyroid glands which sit around the upper pole – damage to which results in hypo-parathyroidism (see below).

Unfortunately sub-total thyroidectomy was in reality really performed because of the nature of the thyroid enlargement in Graves disease making surgery quite challenging.

In most cases the thyroid enlargement of Graves disease results in the upper poles of each thyroid lobe getting bulky and extending superiorly in the neck. Surgery to remove this element is tricky in some patients and particularly with low neck incisions as used to be used almost impossible in some.

Left in-situ remnants of the thyroid can enlarge in the future and cause a recurrence of the Graves disease which is clearly not good as the poor patient then has to have further treatment and potentially have radioactive iodine which is usually something they wished to avoid by having surgery in the first place.

The other issue with sub-total surgery is that it seemed unable to prevent hypocalcaemia and in fact the evidence from large series is that this is a surgeon-dependent complication and not down to the exact nature of the surgery.

Thyroid Surgery

Thyroidectomy requires a general anaesthetic and a stay in hospital, which is normally just overnight.

Access to the neck obviously requires that the surgeon make an incision in the neck. This is made a couple of finger breadths above the top of the breastbone, it is made in a natural skin crease of the neck.

This 'collar incision' is symmetrical even if the thyroid abnormality is only on one side. The incision will usually be 5-6cm in total length although this is increased to give more space for larger goitres and in patients who are significantly overweight.

Most thyroidectomy incisions heal to produce a very satisfactory scar. The skin wound will be closed with a single suture under the skin, which is removed 3-4 days post-operatively, alternatives to this include dissolvable sutures and skin glue.

Possible complications

Most thyroid operations are straightforward and associated with few problems. However all operations carry risks which include postoperative infections (e.g., in the wound or a chest infection), bleeding in the wound and miscellaneous problems due to anaesthesia but these are very rare. Some specific complications of thyroid surgery are discussed below.

Scar: The scar may become relatively thick and red for a few months after the operation before fading to a thin white line. Very rarely some patients develop a thick exaggerated scar but this is uncommon.

Voice change: It is impossible to operate on the neck without producing some change in the voice; fortunately this is not normally detectable.

A specific problem related to thyroid surgery is injury to one or both recurrent laryngeal nerves.

These nerves pass very close to the thyroid gland intertwining with the blood vessels of the gland.

The recurrent nerve controls movement of the vocal cords. Injury to either nerve causes hoarseness and weakness of the voice.

It is quite common for one nerve not to work properly after thyroid surgery due to bruising of the nerve but this recovers over a few days or weeks. The voice is left slightly weak and shouting or raising the voice will be difficult and tiring.

The external laryngeal nerve may also be injured and this results in a weakness in the voice although the sound of the voice is unchanged. Difficulty may be found with the high notes when singing, the voice may tire more easily and the power of the shout is reduced. This nerve is important for people who enjoy singing and in particular for professional singers and in these patients there are surgical strategies to minimize the risk of injury.

Careful surgery reduces the risk of permanent accidental damage to a very low level (<1%) but cannot absolutely eliminate it.

Injury to both recurrent laryngeal nerves is extremely rare but is a serious problem and may require a tracheostomy (tube placed through the neck into the windpipe).

Low blood calcium levels: Patients undergoing surgery to the thyroid gland are at risk of developing a low calcium level if the four tiny parathyroid glands which control the level of calcium in the blood stop working after the operation.

This is termed hypo-parathyroidism.

It is normally possible to identify some if not all of these glands and so avoid a long-term problem. Unfortunately even when the glands have been found and kept they may not function.

If this happens then you will need to take extra calcium and/or vitamin D tablets on a permanent basis. The risk of you needing longterm medication because of a low calcium level is very small indeed (about 1 in 50).

Surgery for Graves disease is slightly more troublesome as the bones are affected by parathyroid disease and in some patients for reasons that are not clearly understood there is a process called "bone hunger" which occurs after surgery.

In bone hunger the bones tend to pull in calcium from the blood exacerbating any fall in calcium levels.

If hypo-parathyroidism develops it can be successfully treated by replacing calcium with tablets and boosting vitamin D levels. In most patients the bone hunger resolves rapidly and any damage to the parathyroid glands recovers in a few weeks or months.

Historically, most unit protocols attempted to withdraw calcium and vitamin D supplements as soon as possible but current evidence is that recovery is best when the supplements are maintained for a few months. The reason for this is unclear but may be because the parathyroid glands can be rested during the period of supplementation and recover better as a result.

Thyroid function: Surgery for Graves disease removes all of the thyroid gland then you will require lifelong replacement of thyroxine. Fortunately this is a straightforward once a day regimen with little requirement for adjusting the dosage. A simple annual blood test to check the dose remains correct for you is all that is required.

Bleeding: Any surgical wound may bleed following the operation. Bleeding in the neck from thyroid surgery is rare (about 1 in 100) but does occur and occasionally results in the need to remove the blood clot requiring a second brief operation usually a few hours after the main surgery.

Bleeding causes swelling in the neck which can obstruct the drainage of venous blood and lymph fluid and as a consequence results in oedema of the tissues of the neck. When this occurs and the swelling involves the mucosal membrances of the airway this leads to airway obstruction.

The emergency treatment of this is to open the wound up and relieve the obstruction to venous drainage – this results in a rapid improvement and the patient can then be taken back to the operating theatre and any remaining blood clot cleared out. Often the source of bleeding is not identified.